The Ultimate Macro Method

A Simple, Step By Step, 21 Day Action Plan
To Following A Macro Diet

»» ———— ««

Nancy Bell

Table of Contents

Introduction

»» ———————— ««

Macros are the common denominator in all nutrition plans; it is finding what balance of macros that gives you the desired results. This book provides you with a strategy to learn how to calculate the macros for your body type, and then follow a day by day method to execute a macro-based diet with a "teach and practice" strategy for 21 days. This hands-on beginner approach allows you to gain a foundation of understanding and sequential experience at which you can build off.

I've coached many people on how to follow a macro diet and what I've learned that no matter what the person's experience with nutrition and following meal plans is, jumping in head first without an understanding of the basic principles, basic guide or strategy to build off of it will always lead to one being overwhelmed, inconsistent and eventually quitting.

This book is straight to the point, a no BS approach to teach principles, strategy, and execute with action. You'll learn how to calculate your macros based on any goal and take action with a simple daily execution plan that allows you to succeed daily and learn through personalized experience along the way.

By the end of the Ultimate Macro Method, you'll feel confident in knowing the quantity of food to eat, what to eat, how to still eat the foods you love while staying "on the plan," and most importantly feel confident and at ease with continuing a macro diet day after day.

What you won't find in this book is a plethora of research and information on the science of macronutrient diets. There is plenty of information on the internet to answer your questions if you want to dig deeper into that. The scientific information is easy to get, but taking action with that information is much harder, which is why most people give up on following a macro diet. I've never come across an action plan to help people be successful (and happy) long term sticking to a macro diet. So, that's the purpose of this book!

How To Use This Book

This book is laid out in a particular order to deliver you information before strategy, incorporating a "teach and practice" method. Read through the starting pages of the book to come up with a personalized plan and use the second half of the book to execute.

As you read through the entire book, you'll find out that there are a few diet strategies to incorporate into a macro diet to "dial in" (for lack of a better term) your macros according to body type(s), leaning out or carb cycling. However, don't let this confuse you with putting together and following through on an initial plan to learn the basics and getting the practice of being able to execute a macro diet in the first place. I purposely have this book laid out in a sequential order to help you avoid doing such a thing, too! You'll find extra fat loss strategies to incorporate into macro dieting at the back of the book and they are there for a reason. Hold off on getting fancy with your macros until you've gone through the method to learn and practice first! Don't worry; you'll gain massive results just by following the method set up for your body type.

Complete the book in this order:

1. Understand the principles and practices of a macro diet.
2. Calculate your macros.
3. Customize macros to your body type.
4. Follow the 21-day plan.

After you've successfully executed the plan and grasp it with comfort, then you can get fancy with your macros if you wish!

Understanding The Principle Of
A Macro Diet

»» ———————————— ««

First and foremost, "What is a macro?" Macro is short for "macronutrients." These are our three main food groups, proteins, carbohydrates, and fat. In terms of fitness and weight loss, these macros make up a guide for nutrition plans to achieve fat loss, build lean muscle and increase metabolism. Macro diets require you to consume a suggested amount of grams of proteins, carbohydrates and fats, so it's important to utilize a food log of some sort. There are many strategies to change your body composition and lower body fat. However, simply starting a suggested macro-based diet for your body type can also provide a ton of benefit for nourishing your body properly, eating the right type of calories for your body, and ultimately learning how your body responds to foods.

Macro diets are set up on suggested ratios of macros for different body types. Research shows that each body type utilizes these macronutrients differently. Therefore, following any given macro diet may not necessarily give the results you are looking for. It's important to follow a macro plan suggested for your specific body type to achieve the best results.

While this method is extremely successful, understand that the suggested ratios only gives an individual a basic starting point. Each body type is unique. Various health and lifestyle aspects factor in. For best results, I recommend eating a low sugar, whole food diet 85% of the time. Assure you're getting the proper amount of calories (deficit/surplus) concerning your desired goal. Allow your body 7+ hours of rest per night and be sure you're getting an adequate amount of water as hydration is key for a fully functioning body. If ever you reach a point of plateau and you've ruled out adequate calorie consumption, consider taking a look at a possible "secondary" body type or carb cycle to tweak your macros, which I'll go over in more detail further in the book. Once macros have been set, always allow at minimum two weeks of consistent follow through to see results before adjusting.

The Long-term Practice Of A Macro Diet

Often people fear how this affects them in the long run if they were to stop following a particular diet like this or stop being as regimented. The big picture idea of learning a macro-based diet is allowing the person to create awareness with their body so they understand how food affects it. Whether that's from a physiological or physique standpoint, once a person learns the basics and builds off it, they'll grasp an awareness of 1.) how much they're actually consuming in a given meal, 2.) how their body responds to eating meals/foods made up of such and 3.) how a certain balance of calories/macros will affect them today or two weeks from now.

Once you learn the basics and understand the best balance of macros for your body type, you can then move into a more flexible lifestyle without losing your progress.

Over time, after practicing a regimented diet, you become very attuned to eating in a way that makes you feel your best. So just because you started a macro diet, doesn't mean you have to be extremely regimented with your food and log your food forever, but if followed long enough, you'll create enough awareness and knowledge for your body to continue living healthy and sustainable habits in alignment with your nutritional and fitness goals.

Calculating Your Macros

In order to calculate your macros, there are a few important numbers you need to know about your body to give you the most accurate starting point. You need to calculate your:

1. BMR (Basal Metabolic Rate - *how many calories you burn just living and breathing*).
2. TDEE (Total Daily Energy Expenditure – *how much energy you burn, including exercise and daily activity*).
3. Total Daily Calorie Intake Goal incorporating a deficit/surplus of calories for your fitness/weight loss goal.
4. Macros suggested to your body type.

To get the calculations all in one place, visit tdeecalculator.net. This site will automatically give you calculations based on your age, weight, height and level of activity. What you want to understand first is your "maintenance" calories. *(See next page)*

TDEE Calculator

YOUR STATS

bodyfat

You are a 31 y/o Female ∨ who is 125 lbs and 5ft 3in ∨ with Moderate Exercise ∨   % Re-Calculate

optional

You left the body fat percentage field blank. A more accurate formula is used to estimate your TDEE when you know it. To learn your body fat percentage with calipers, click here

Your Maintenance Calories	Based on your stats, the best estimate for your maintenance calories is **1,939** calories per day based on the Mifflin-St Jeor Formula, which is widely known to be the most accurate. The table below shows the difference if you were to have selected a different activity level.	
1,939 calories per day	Basal Metabolic Rate	1,251 calories per day
	Sedentary	1,501 calories per day
	Light Exercise	1,720 calories per day
13,575 calories per week	**Moderate Exercise**	**1,939 calories per day**
	Heavy Exercise	2,158 calories per day
	Athlete	2,377 calories per day

Now, you can add or subtract the appropriate amount of calories based on your fitness/weight loss goal using the suggestions below:

- **Weight Loss:** Generally speaking, there are about 3,500 calories in a pound. Most dieticians recommend eating a deficit of anywhere between 500-1,000 calories a day. *(i.e., looking at a TDEE of 2,200, if you aimed for 1,700 calories per day, you'd be eating at a 500 calorie deficient. This would put you at approximately losing 1 pound per week.)*

- **Maintenance:** Consume the same amount of calories of your BMR + TDEE.

- **Muscle Gain:** You need to supply the body with a surplus of calories to generate new, lean, muscle mass tissue. Just like fat, a pound of muscle equals 3500 calories. So, in order to safely and effectively gain muscle, you need to increase your total calorie intake by a minimum of 3500 calories per week. That works out to about 500 extra calories per day. So, add 500 calories + BMR + TDEE to get your total daily calorie goal. It's important to understand that when adopting a muscle-gain diet, you are going to acquire some fat—this is normal. A one-to-two-pound a week weight gain goal should average 75% muscle and 25% fat. Once you've reached your desired muscle gains, then you can work to trim unwanted fat off slowly.

Customizing Macros To Your Body Type

»» ———————— ««

Ultimately, your genes determine your body type. Each person is unique and stores body fat in different areas. In most cases, fat is not evenly distributed; some people gain weight in their midsection and arms, while others gain it in their butt and thighs.

Your body shape is also affected by hormones. For example, research shows that the hormone cortisol is stored in the midsection, and estrogen or progesterone are stored more in the lower abdomen. It is always important to take general health into account as your body transforms and you make adjustments to your macros and nutrient intake.

There are three main body types when referring to macronutrients for your body: ectomorph, mesomorph, and endomorph. *(*See images on page 12)*

a. **Ectomorph:** The body is straight up and down with not much of a defined waist. Shoulders and hips are about the same width. An ectomorph is naturally skinny with longer limbs. The shoulders, waist and hips are almost the same widths. They typically have a harder time building muscle. Ectomorphs have a high carb tolerance.

b. **Mesomorph:** The shoulders and hips are nearly the same widths apart and the waist is smaller. The upper and lower body are opposing triangles facing in. A mesomorph is naturally muscular and athletic. The shoulders and hips are about the same width. They can build muscle easily. Mesomorphs have a moderate carb tolerance.

c. **Endomorph:** Has shoulders that are broader than their hips. The hips and legs don't accumulate excess fat, as the waist up typically does. Endomorphs are naturally broad and thick. Shoulders are wider than the hips. They can build muscle fairly well, however losing fat takes more diligent work with nutrition. Endomorphs have a low carb tolerance.

Body Type	Macronutrients	Visual
Ectomorph	Protein: 35% Carbs: 45% Fats: 20%	
Mesomorph	Protein: 30% Carbs: 40% Fats: 30%	
Endomorph	Protein: 35% Carbs: 30% Fats: 35%	

Each body type has a suggested percentage of each macronutrient to eat because of how the body type metabolizes food and stores fat. As I mentioned earlier, you may have a secondary body type (a combination of two body types), that you may need to consider if you're not seeing results with following the macros of one of the three main body types.

Once you have determined your body type, you need to take your total daily caloric intake and figure out how many grams you need of each macronutrient. I will show you how to set this up in My Fitness Pal in the next chapter if you want to skip the math, but I do think it's a helpful tool to understand how to calculate these numbers, so I'll walk you through an example.

To calculate your macros manually, you need to know how many calories are in 1 gram of each macronutrient. Protein holds 4 calories per gram, carbohydrates holds 4 calories per gram, and fats holds 9 calories per gram. Using this information, you'll take your total daily calories multiplied by each percentage for each macronutrient group, and then divide it by the number of calories per gram for that given macronutrient to get your daily macros.

To give an example, I walk you through a scenario to set up a person's macros customized to their body type below.

Example:

Jane's total daily calorie intake comes to 1,939 maintenance calories. She wants to lose 4 pounds per month, and about 1 pound per week. Her goal is to be in a deficit of 3,500 calories each week to reach her 1lb weight loss goal per week. This brings Jane to require a 500 calorie deficit each day. To be in a deficit, she can exercise to burn calories or cut her calories back. For this example, let's say on average, Jane exercises 3-5 times a week and burns about 400 calories per workout, putting her at 1,539 calories. For Jane to align with her calorie deficit, she needs to meet her weight loss goal; she needs to cut back or burn another 100 calories per day. Jane decides to cut her daily caloric intake by 100 more calories to make up the difference, putting her at 1,439 calories per day.

Now that Jane knows what her calorie intake goal should be to meet her goal, she needs to customize it to her body type. Jane is a mesomorph, so she calculates her 1,439 daily calories according to the suggested mesomorph macronutrient ratios:

30% Protein:

- 1,439(total calories) x .30 (protein) = 432 calories (needed daily for protein intake)

    432 calories / 4 calories (4 calories in 1g protein) = **108g of protein needed each day**

30% Fat:

- 1,439(total calories) x .30 (fat) = 432 calories (needed daily for fat intake)

    432 calories / 9 calories (9 calories in 1g fat) =

    48g of fat needed each day

40% Carbohydrates:

- 1,439(total calories) x .40 (carbs) = 576 calories (needed daily for carbohydrate intake)

    576 calories / 4 calories (4 calories in 1g carbs) = **144g of protein needed each day**

Jane's daily macros to lose 1lb per week are:

- Protein: 108g
- Fats: 48g
- Carbs: 144g

Fill in the blank table below to calculate your macros.

Jane's Example:

TDEE Calculator Maintenance Calories			1,939
Deficit/Surplus			-500
Add or subtract exercise and food calories to get your final total daily caloric intake	(-) Exercise _-400_		(-/+) Calories _-100_
Total Daily Calorie Intake Goal			1,439
Body Type _Mesomorph_	P: 30%	F: 30%	C: 40%
Protein 1,439cals x . 30% = 432 cals / 4			= 108 grams
Fat 1,439cals x . 30% = 432 cals / 9			= 48 grams
Carbs 1,439cals x . 40% = 576 cals / 4			= 144 grams

My Macros

TDEE Calculator Maintenance Calories			
Deficit/Surplus			
Add or subtract exercise and food calories to get your final total daily caloric intake	(-) Exercise _____		(-/+) Calories _____
Total Daily Calorie Intake Goal			
Body Type _____	P:____%	F: ____%	C: ____%
Protein _____cals x .___% = ____cals/4			= grams
Fat_____cals x .___% = ____cals/4			= grams
Carbs_____cals x .___% = ____cals/4			= grams

How To Read and Track Macronutrients

》 ———————— 《

When you're following a macro diet, you're eating your meals/foods based on the grams in each macronutrient. Therefore, you need to count the total number of grams you have for proteins, carbohydrates and fats to reach your daily calorie intake goal. To "count macros"/grams, simply read the nutrition label on foods. It's important to pay attention to serving size, so you know how many grams of each protein, carb, and fat are in one serving. The following picture is an example of what to look at:

Serving sizes are typically measured "as is." Some labels will

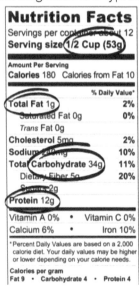

specify dry/mixed. In this example of pancake mix, a serving size is 1/2c dry mix. Anything you add into your mix or have with the meal would also need to be separately looked at and added to count your daily macros.

*Most foods are generally measured or weighed after cooking. Most foods have 2-3 ways to measure; cups/ounces or grams.

16

Most whole foods do not have a nutrition label; however, if you utilize the app "My Fitness Pal" to track your macros, you can scan the barcode into your diary to get the nutritional value of the food. Google is always a good resource too.

When tracking your macros, you can keep track by paper and pen, adding up each food's macros or you utilize an app to do the math for you. I've found "My Fitness Pal" (MFP) to be the most user-friendly app with an expansive database of foods on the market. Using an app is less time consuming than calculating by hand. I've included simple instructions for setting up your MFP app in this chapter to help you get started with tracking. If you can set up your MFP app before you begin logging, it will drastically help with time and unnecessary feelings of overwhelm. I highly recommend setting this up *before* you begin tracking your foods, including scanning your top frequent 15 foods.

Setting Up My Fitness Pal With Your Customized Macros (using an iOS)

1. Go to your iOS app store, download "My Fitness Pal."
2. Create an account or sign in.
3. Upon logging in, it will bring you to your "home" page, showing a newsfeed.
4. On the bottom right, click on "more…"
5. In this menu, select "goals."
6. Under the section "Nutrition Goals," select "Calorie, Carb, Protein, and Fat Goals."
7. Next, select "Calories."
8. Type in the daily recommended calorie intake for your goals, and select the check mark to set it.

9. Then select "Carbohydrates." This brings up percentages of each macro to customize your body type as you found on page 12. Select the check mark once you've input your percentages.

You do not need to adjust percentages according to "grams" to get started. You can utilize the free version of this app. If/when you dial in your macros more particularly from either adjusting to a secondary body type or carb cycle, you may need to get the upgraded premium version, however, you can accomplish a lot on the free version.

How To Log Food in My Fitness Pal

Click on "diary" on the bottom menu. Here you can select "add food" for the meal you are logging. After tapping on this, I suggest using the barcode scanner to the right of the search bar to scan the particular food in rather than trying to find your food and brand of food in the search menu. If the barcode doesn't work, then use your best judgement and search methods to find the food that you're trying to log in using your search bar. *Tip: Scan/add your top frequent 15 foods into a day of your diary for ease. (See page 23)*

Adjust Meal Names in My Fitness Pal

I'm including this instruction because I found it very helpful. Most nutrition plan recommends eating 4-6 meals a day and it's more confusing to call these meals by "breakfast," "lunch," "dinner" and "snacks," so I personally label mine "meal 1," "meal 2," "meal 3," "meal 4," "meal 5," and "meal 6."

To adjust the meal names, click on "more…" on the bottom menu. Select "Settings." Next select "Diary Settings." Then select "Customized Meal Names," and from there, you can label your meals. Use the check mark on the top right corner to save.

Viewing Your Macros To Plan Your Meals

I utilize the "nutrient" tool of each meal to see where I'm currently at with my macros to plan or create my next meal. To view this, select "Diary" on the bottom menu. Next, at the top of the screen where it lists "Calories Remaining," your calorie "goal" – "food" + "exercise" = "Remaining" is listed. Tap on "Remaining" calories and it will bring you to a screen that lists "Calories." "Nutrients" and "Macros." Then, tap on "Nutrients." Here this screen will show your current "Total" (what you have consumed/logged so far), your "Goal" (what you have set customized to daily goal), and "Left" (what you have left to consume for the day). When I go to prepare a meal, I look to see what I have left and divide that number out by the number of meals I am planning to prepare the rest of the day to come up with a target for the meal I'm going to eat at that time. This is where it helps to input meals you already have planned so you can eat accordingly for unplanned meals.

Adding Recipes or Food Not Found In Search Bar

When I can't find a food in the search bar or it won't scan with the barcode feature (typically whole foods or off-brand labels), you can either input the macros from the nutrition label, or from what you find with a google search. Go to your Diary. Select "Add Food." At the top of the screen, select "+" From there select "Create Food." Input the Brand Name, Description, Serving Size, and Servings Per Container (or number of servings). Select the arrow at the top to continue. Input the information you have from the nutrition label or have found using google search. Select the check mark to save. You can utilize this feature when you combine ingredients to make a particular or frequent meal/recipe too.

Other Features To Use In My Fitness Pal

Aside from features, I've already walked you through other great features to utilize in this app, such as the progress tracking, diary sharing (accountability from friends or coaches), and the home feature where you can find fitness tips and new recipes.

I do not sync up my devices with the My Fitness Pal app as it will add "exercise" calories to your daily consumption. You've already calculated that in by adding in your "TDEE" to get your daily caloric intake.

Practice!

Grab a piece of paper and pen and write down the macros of the foods you had for breakfast, including condiments and cooking oils. For simplicity, just write down a serving size if you didn't measure. Add each macro up (protein, carb, fat). This is what your macros totaled for breakfast. To get your daily macros, you would just do this for each meal. Pretty simple, but it can get overwhelming and, in some cases, tricky, so let's keep moving on.

Getting Acquainted!

Now that we've covered the "set up" phase, it's time to take action with the steps that are going to help you be successful by learning through practice and hands on experience. DO NOT skip this chapter as this is one of the most helpful tools to learning and following through on a macro diet. This is the phase that eliminates the overwhelm and brings simplicity!

First, we are going to make a list of your Top 15 Frequent Foods. We all have foods we turn to the most on a daily basis, and it helps to get familiar with what these are and learn their macros to gain insight on what adjustments you may need to make to keep macro life simple.

On the next page, go through the top 15 foods you eat on a daily basis and write down what each of the macros are. For you to become aware of how much protein, fat and carbs in each will be helpful for you to know when navigating your meal choices. Pay attention to how many grams of macros that are in each food and think about how having those particular foods will impact your daily goal.

If you plan to utilize the MFP app (which I highly recommend), then this is also a good time to scan these 15 foods into a day of your diary. Once they are scanned in your diary, you'll be able to "quick add" them and find them at the top of the diary's food list. This will be helpful when you start tracking.

Top 15 Frequent Foods

Food	Fat Grams	Carb Grams	Protein Grams

Now you can take a baseline measurement of where you naturally fall with your caloric intake and macros by logging one full day of food. Look back on a day to track/log the food you ate to get a realistic view of where you fall in alignment with your new macro goals. You can do this by writing down or logging in the MFP app what you ate yesterday or log the foods you eat today (what you would naturally eat). If you cannot remember or don't want to spend a day tracking to get this step done, you can also make an example meal plan day of what you typically eat in a day. Any of these will work for you to get an idea of what your daily intake currently looks like. If your food varies quite a bit day to day, then do this for a couple of days incorporating the different foods. I provided a couple of food logs on the next two pages if you choose to do it manually.

Once you have logged your food for a day or two, take a look at your total daily grams for each macronutrient. See where your daily total measures with regards to your new macro goals. Are you "over" or "under" grams in any of the categories? Did one meal have significantly more grams (more calories) all together than others? Did any particular meal consume the majority of one of your macros? Did you feel full after your meals?

If you're using MFP, reference page 19, section "Viewing Your Macros To Plan Your Meals," to quickly see your daily total.

Breakfast

Food	Fat	Carbs	Protein
Total			

Lunch

Food	Fat	Carbs	Protein
Total			

Supper

Food	Fat	Carbs	Protein
Total			

Snack(s)

Food	Fat	Carbs	Protein
Total			

Daily Total

Food	Fat	Carbs	Protein

Breakfast

Food	Fat	Carbs	Protein
Total			

Lunch

Food	Fat	Carbs	Protein
Total			

Supper

Food	Fat	Carbs	Protein
Total			

Snack(s)

Food	Fat	Carbs	Protein
Total			

Daily Total

Food	Fat	Carbs	Protein

Elimination Process

Now that you can see at a glance what your Top 15 Frequent Foods are and what daily food looks like for you, you can get a better idea of which foods you can either eliminate, eat more of or swap out for another food choice. Knowing which foods hinder or help you reach your daily macro goal allows you to plan easier. It doesn't mean you need to eliminate certain foods altogether or get uncomfortably full eating multiple servings of others; but it does show you which foods you may need to strategize more around to have or not have while still reaching your daily macro goal. This introduces you to the concept of "flexible" eating or in other words, "you can have your cake and eat it too"!

Flexible Eating

The concept of flexible eating is to be able to eat foods that are "not so clean" if they fit within your macros for the day. For instance, you want to eat mac n' cheese or have a chocolate bar, you can! You would just make room in your macros for the day. This will allow you to not worry about going off plan, feel guilty, or have to eliminate your favorite foods altogether. I recommend finding a balance of 85% clean and 15% "un-clean" so that you can nourish your body and still set yourself up to get results because at the end of the day, the value of the calories still matters. The more whole foods you eat, the better your results. You will also stay satiated longer when eating whole foods as opposed to processed or refined foods that leave you feeling hungry or don't satisfy you. As you learn to track macros, you'll quickly find how foods affect you and will become aware of what works well or doesn't work for you too.

Weighing vs. Measuring

When tracking macros, you need to measure or weigh your foods to make sure you're getting the correct serving amount. I suggest buying a digital food scale, a liquid measuring cup, a set of dry measuring cups and a set of measuring spoons. You'll use the food scale the most when eating whole foods as their contents are best measured by ounces or grams in weight. Boxed or canned foods, grains and condiments can easily be measured by using measuring cups or spoons, but again for best accuracy, use a food scale. Liquids are best measured with liquid measuring cups as the amount differs from a dry measuring cup.

When weighing your foods, always weigh the item you have the food in first so you can subtract that once you have the food on the scale too. If you have the ability to measure your foods use a digital scale as much as you can, there can be quite a variance in comparison to measuring in cups/ounces versus a digital scale measuring in grams/ounces. Here's an example on the next page:

Nutrition Facts

About 15 servings per container

Serving size   1/2 cup mix (59g)

Amount per serving

Calories   210

	% Daily Value*
Total Fat 1.5g	**2%**
Saturated Fat 0g	**0%**
Trans Fat 0g	
Cholesterol 0mg	**0%**
Sodium 660mg	**29%**
Total Carbohydrate 45g	**16%**
Dietary Fiber < 1g	**3%**
Total Sugars 11g	
Includes 10g Added Sugars	**20%**
Protein 4g	

Vitamin D 0mcg	0%
Calcium 80mg	6%
Iron 1.9mg	10%
Potassium 60mg	0%

* The % Daily Value (DV) tells you how much a nutrient in a serving of food contributes to a daily diet. 2,000 calories a day is used for general nutrition advice.

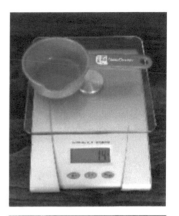

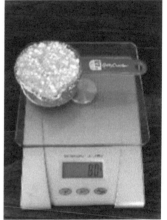

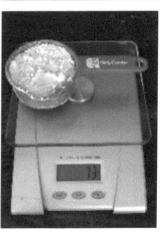

See the serving size of this pancake mix. Weigh the item you are weighing foods in (Photo #1)

See the difference between 1/2c measured (photo #2) and 59g weighed (Photo #3) *According to the food label to the left.

Food Preparation

When it comes to food prep for tracking macros, I highly recommend cooking your proteins, fats and carbohydrates separately so that you can accurately measure each before you eat them or combine them to make a dish (i.e chicken rice bowl). As you get more comfortable with tracking, then tackle making "recipes" with combined ingredients.

If you have "go-to" meal prep foods on your Top 15 Frequent Food list, and you want to cook in bulk, then follow the steps below to track your macros in the recipe. After you do it once, you won't need to do it again unless you change the number of servings.

1. Write down the macros for a serving of each ingredient (or utilize the "Create a Recipe" function in MFP app to scan and calculate for you).
2. Multiply your ingredients to the number of servings you want to prepare.
3. Write the multiplied macros for each ingredient.
4. Divide the macros by the number of servings you have prepared.

If you have a simple recipe with few ingredients to track, this is a quick and easy task. However, if you are trying to make your recipe have a balance of macros for your meal target, it can become overwhelming to add, take away or reduce ingredients to hit your goal. This is where I'd suggest making macros simple by keeping the proteins, carbs and fats separate, atleast for the majority of your meals.

In addition to food prep suggestions, I highly recommend always having a few "grab and go" options on hand, whether it is a protein bar, meal replacement drink, or banana and yogurt. There are some days where these quick "grab and go" meals will come in handy. You might find this to a "must" to keeping macro life simple, too.

The Method: Building A Foundation

》》 ———————— 《《

Now that you have already set your macro goal when you calculated how much you need to be consuming in grams of each macronutrient, you will need to make smaller goals within that. To set yourself up for success, I highly recommend breaking down your daily macro goal to create small "meal goals" to help you end your day on plan. You can do this by dividing your daily macro goal by the number of meals you eat. I'll use Jane's macros from page 15 as an example.

We know her daily macro goal is to consume 108g protein, 48g fat, and 144g carbs. She plans to eat 5 small meals a day. If she divides her total grams of each macronutrient by 5, this will give her a target for each meal.

Jane's Macros (Daily Macro Goal):
108g (protein) / 5 = 22g
48g (fats) / 5 = 10g
144g (carbohydrates) / 5 = 29g
Jane's macro target for each meal is to consume 22g of protein, 10g of fat and 29g of carbs.

Using the math equation (Daily Macro/number of meals), calculate your macro target for your meals below:

My Macro Meal Goal

Fat:	Grams
Carb:	Grams
Protein:	Grams

The Method: Week 1

»» ———————— ««

During week 1, you're going to be building a foundation to ease into tracking your macros. After this week, you'll have a baseline structure of meals and foods you can always rely on that fall within your macro target for meals.

The focus of this week is to learn "go-to," reliable and preferred meals with balanced macros for you that you can incorporate into your "full time" macro plan with ease and comfort. Once you establish and finish this step, you'll always have this foundation to fall onto if you ever get off track, or decide to have a period of time to not aggressively track macros. Also, by knowing these "go-to" meals, you'll have a safety net for when you don't have food prepared, you're on the go, or if you decide to not aggressively track for a day, this will bring comfort knowing you have options that are balanced and on target.

This week, you will track two meals and one macronutrient group to start building this foundation. Each day you will plan for the next day. You can do this by taking a look at your "Top 15 Frequent Foods" list on page 23 and pick out foods that will add up to your "meal goal" as you calculated on page 33. It's okay to be over/under within 5 grams of each macro. If you find out that the foods you picked don't add up to your macro meal goal, then consider adding an additional serving, or a partial serving of another food you frequently eat. For example, if you typically eat one slice of bread for breakfast which gives you about 19g of carbohydrates, but your target is 32g, then you might consider adding half of an apple or another half piece of toast, or adding jelly to your toast to make up the difference in carbohydrates. Another example, if you frequently have egg whites and toast, but now realize you don't have any fat included, you can now add a condiment by cooking your eggs with olive oil, or add in some avocado to meet the macros for that meal. It is up to you however you want to make up your macro's for each meal; just be sure it's within 5 grams of each (over/under) macronutrient for your "Macro Meal Goal."

Next, track these two meals in your MFP app or on the food log I've provided on the next page. These will now be two meals planned for the next day.

Finally, on the day of, you will begin learning and practicing tracking macro's in a more unprepared "as you go" manner. This week you will start with only tracking proteins in addition to your two planned meals. Each meal you will aim to hit your "meal goal" for protein by weighing or measuring your protein servings. 2 meals are already planned for, so that leaves the remainder of your meals left to measure at the time of each meal (or prep/pack it if you're not going to be home). For example, if you planned two midday meals for your workday, you will need to measure your morning and evening protein servings. I suggest having foods you would normally eat, just measure or weigh out the serving size to hit your goal. Again, use the MFP app or food logs provided to track the protein macro's you consume.

This week you will not worry about tracking carbohydrates and fats outside of your planned meals. This week's focus is practicing towards your two planned meals and tracking/aiming and learning foods for your protein goal for all other meals. Eat fats and carbs as you normally would. Utilize the food logs in the rest of this chapter (or MFP app) to track your foods. See an example day on the next page.

Summary of Week 1 Plan:

Plan 2 meals

Track Protein for all other meals

Jane's Food Log Examples:

Meal 1 -Morning Snack (Planned Meal #1)

Food	Fat	Carb	Protein
Protein Bar – Blueberry Cobbler	8g	24g	20g

Meal 2 – Lunch (Planned Meal #2)

Food	Fat	Carb	Protein
4oz. 93/7 beef	8g	0g	23g
Hamburger Bun	1g	28g	3g
½ cucumber	0g	4g	0g
Mustard	0g	0g	0g
1 tbsp. Ketchup	0g	4g	0g
Lettuce Leaf	0g	0g	0g
3 sliced pickles	0g	0g	0g

*Note: There is no need to log foods that have 0's for macro's, this is just an example. Fibrous vegetables such as cucumbers are optional to track, dependent upon your need for accuracy.

Meal 3 -Breakfast (Protein)

Food	Fat	Carb	Protein
1/2c. Cottage Cheese	2.5g	5g	12g

Meal 4 – Afternoon Snack (Protein)

Food	Fat	Carb	Protein
Protein Shake w/ water	1g	3g	23g

Meal 5 - Supper (Protein)

Food	Fat	Carb	Protein
4oz Chicken Breast	1.5g	0g	26g

	Fat	Carb	Protein
Daily Total	**22g**	**68g**	**107g**

*Jane hit her protein macro goal falling 1g short (Protein goal: 108g) She is disregarding fats and carbs this week.

**By labeling meals with "numbers," no specific order is needed.

DAY 1

Meal 1 - (Planned Meal #1)

Food	Fat	Carb	Protein

Meal 2 – (Planned Meal #2)

Food	Fat	Carb	Protein

Meal 3 - (Protein)

Food	Fat	Carb	Protein

Meal 4 – (Protein)

Food	Fat	Carb	Protein

Meal 5 - (Protein)

Food	Fat	Carb	Protein

Meal 6 - (Protein)

Food	Fat	Carb	Protein

Daily Total	Fat	Carb	Protein

DAY 2

Meal 1 - (Planned Meal #1)

Food	Fat	Carb	Protein

Meal 2 – (Planned Meal #2)

Food	Fat	Carb	Protein

Meal 3 - (Protein)

Food	Fat	Carb	Protein

Meal 4 – (Protein)

Food	Fat	Carb	Protein

Meal 5 - (Protein)

Food	Fat	Carb	Protein

Meal 6 - (Protein)

Food	Fat	Carb	Protein

Daily Total	Fat	Carb	Protein

DAY 3

Meal 1 - (Planned Meal #1)

Food	Fat	Carb	Protein

Meal 2 – (Planned Meal #2)

Food	Fat	Carb	Protein

Meal 3 - (Protein)

Food	Fat	Carb	Protein

Meal 4 – (Protein)

Food	Fat	Carb	Protein

Meal 5 - (Protein)

Food	Fat	Carb	Protein

Meal 6 - (Protein)

Food	Fat	Carb	Protein

Daily Total	Fat	Carb	Protein

DAY 4

Meal 1 - (Planned Meal #1)

Food	Fat	Carb	Protein

Meal 2 – (Planned Meal #2)

Food	Fat	Carb	Protein

Meal 3 - (Protein)

Food	Fat	Carb	Protein

Meal 4 – (Protein)

Food	Fat	Carb	Protein

Meal 5 - (Protein)

Food	Fat	Carb	Protein

Meal 6 - (Protein)

Food	Fat	Carb	Protein

Daily Total	Fat	Carb	Protein

DAY 5

Meal 1 - (Planned Meal #1)

Food	Fat	Carb	Protein

Meal 2 – (Planned Meal #2)

Food	Fat	Carb	Protein

Meal 3 - (Protein)

Food	Fat	Carb	Protein

Meal 4 – (Protein)

Food	Fat	Carb	Protein

Meal 5 - (Protein)

Food	Fat	Carb	Protein

Meal 6 - (Protein)

Food	Fat	Carb	Protein

Daily Total	Fat	Carb	Protein

DAY 6

Meal 1 - (Planned Meal #1)

Food	Fat	Carb	Protein

Meal 2 – (Planned Meal #2)

Food	Fat	Carb	Protein

Meal 3 - (Protein)

Food	Fat	Carb	Protein

Meal 4 – (Protein)

Food	Fat	Carb	Protein

Meal 5 - (Protein)

Food	Fat	Carb	Protein

Meal 6 - (Protein)

Food	Fat	Carb	Protein

Daily Total	Fat	Carb	Protein

DAY 7

Meal 1 - (Planned Meal #1)

Food	Fat	Carb	Protein

Meal 2 – (Planned Meal #2)

Food	Fat	Carb	Protein

Meal 3 - (Protein)

Food	Fat	Carb	Protein

Meal 4 – (Protein)

Food	Fat	Carb	Protein

Meal 5 - (Protein)

Food	Fat	Carb	Protein

Meal 6 - (Protein)

Food	Fat	Carb	Protein

Daily Total	Fat	Carb	Protein

The Method: Week 2

»» ———————— ««

Week 2 is very similar to week 1. This week you'll continue to focus on practicing meal prep for at least two meals just like in week one and continue to track and aim for your protein macros each meal. Remember, each of these planned meals meets your macro "meal goal" for each meal (daily total divided by # of meals). These two meals are planned, on track and a preference of yours so no extra energy should be spent worrying about them to keep your focus on the other 2-4 meals that are not planned out for you. I highly recommend you continue to eat the same two planned meals you've now established for simplicity.

This week, you'll add tracking fats in addition to protein. You've now established which proteins and serving sizes get you to your macro meal goal for your protein intake, so now you can narrow in on these proteins to find where fats can fit in. Typically, protein servings will already include your fat serving, so it's important to find which of these proteins in your diet already include this or don't include it. If you're eating lean proteins, you'll have flexibility to add in cooking oils or condiments. However, if you're eating 93/7 or fattier meats, you'll lose some flexibility in some meals. Again, divide your total daily fat goal by the number of meals you'll be eating to get your "meal goal." Aim to get this amount of fat per meal to land on track with your total daily macro goal.

Summary of Week 2 Plan:
Plan 2 meals
Track Protein and fats for all other meals.
See food log notes below Jane's example food log.

Jane's Food Log Examples:

Meal 1 -Morning Snack (Planned Meal #1)

Food	Fat	Carb	Protein
Protein Bar – Blueberry Cobbler	8g	24g	20g

Meal 2 – Lunch (Planned Meal #2)

Food	Fat	Carb	Protein
4oz. 93/7 beef	8g	0g	23g
Hamburger Bun, lettuce, pickles	1g	28g	3g
½ cucumber	0g	4g	0g
1 tbsp. Ketchup & Mustard	0g	4g	0g

*Foods with 0 macros were removed to show a realistic food log.

Meal 3 -Breakfast (Protein & Fat)

Food	Fat	Carb	Protein
2 eggs w/ yolk, 3oz egg whites	10g	0g	10g
3oz egg whites	0g	0g	12g

Meal 4 – Afternoon Snack (Protein & Fat)

Food	Fat	Carb	Protein
Protein Shake	2g	4g	22g
PB2 w/ chocolate	1g	6g	4g
Unsweetened Vanilla Alm. Milk	1g	2.5g	1g

Meal 5 - Supper (Protein & Fat)

Food	Fat	Carb	Protein
4oz 99/1 Ground Turkey	2g	0g	26g
1 slice cheese	6g	0g	5g
Daily Total	39g	70g	127g

Jane missed her daily macro goal, falling 19g over on her protein macros. Jane's macro goal: F: 48g, P:108g. She may consider reducing the amount of protein at one or two of her meals to fall closer to her daily macro goal. She may realize that her fat was just on the edge of falling short, so she may add in a little extra fat with one meal. This week she is disregarding her carb goal, only focusing on reaching her protein and fat goals.

DAY 8

Meal 1 - (Planned Meal #1)

Food	Fat	Carb	Protein

Meal 2 – (Planned Meal #2)

Food	Fat	Carb	Protein

Meal 3 - (Protein)

Food	Fat	Carb	Protein

Meal 4 – (Protein)

Food	Fat	Carb	Protein

Meal 5 - (Protein)

Food	Fat	Carb	Protein

Meal 6 - (Protein)

Food	Fat	Carb	Protein

Daily Total	Fat	Carb	Protein

DAY 9

Meal 1 - (Planned Meal #1)

Food	Fat	Carb	Protein

Meal 2 – (Planned Meal #2)

Food	Fat	Carb	Protein

Meal 3 - (Protein)

Food	Fat	Carb	Protein

Meal 4 – (Protein)

Food	Fat	Carb	Protein

Meal 5 - (Protein)

Food	Fat	Carb	Protein

Meal 6 - (Protein)

Food	Fat	Carb	Protein

Daily Total	Fat	Carb	Protein

DAY 10

Meal 1 - (Planned Meal #1)

Food	Fat	Carb	Protein

Meal 2 – (Planned Meal #2)

Food	Fat	Carb	Protein

Meal 3 - (Protein)

Food	Fat	Carb	Protein

Meal 4 – (Protein)

Food	Fat	Carb	Protein

Meal 5 - (Protein)

Food	Fat	Carb	Protein

Meal 6 - (Protein)

Food	Fat	Carb	Protein

Daily Total	Fat	Carb	Protein

DAY 11

Meal 1 - (Planned Meal #1)

Food	Fat	Carb	Protein

Meal 2 – (Planned Meal #2)

Food	Fat	Carb	Protein

Meal 3 - (Protein)

Food	Fat	Carb	Protein

Meal 4 – (Protein)

Food	Fat	Carb	Protein

Meal 5 - (Protein)

Food	Fat	Carb	Protein

Meal 6 - (Protein)

Food	Fat	Carb	Protein

Daily Total	Fat	Carb	Protein

DAY 12

Meal 1 - (Planned Meal #1)

Food	Fat	Carb	Protein

Meal 2 – (Planned Meal #2)

Food	Fat	Carb	Protein

Meal 3 - (Protein)

Food	Fat	Carb	Protein

Meal 4 – (Protein)

Food	Fat	Carb	Protein

Meal 5 - (Protein)

Food	Fat	Carb	Protein

Meal 6 - (Protein)

Food	Fat	Carb	Protein

Daily Total	Fat	Carb	Protein

DAY 13

Meal 1 - (Planned Meal #1)

Food	Fat	Carb	Protein

Meal 2 – (Planned Meal #2)

Food	Fat	Carb	Protein

Meal 3 - (Protein)

Food	Fat	Carb	Protein

Meal 4 – (Protein)

Food	Fat	Carb	Protein

Meal 5 - (Protein)

Food	Fat	Carb	Protein

Meal 6 - (Protein)

Food	Fat	Carb	Protein

Daily Total	Fat	Carb	Protein

DAY 14

Meal 1 - (Planned Meal #1)

Food	Fat	Carb	Protein

Meal 2 – (Planned Meal #2)

Food	Fat	Carb	Protein

Meal 3 - (Protein)

Food	Fat	Carb	Protein

Meal 4 – (Protein)

Food	Fat	Carb	Protein

Meal 5 - (Protein)

Food	Fat	Carb	Protein

Meal 6 - (Protein)

Food	Fat	Carb	Protein

Daily Total	Fat	Carb	Protein

The Method: Week 3

»» —————————— ««

Week 3, you'll continue to have at least two planned meals, and by now, you've most likely established one to two other meal options that you prefer and frequently eat. This week add in one more planned meal for simplicity and ease as you begin tracking and learning another macro, carbohydrates during this week. Typically, this 3rd planned meal most easily ends up being breakfast or a snack prior to, after supper or a time frame in the day in which there's not much time to make a small meal.

Continue tracking all three macros for three planned meals, hitting your "meal goal." This week you'll also calculate your carb "meal goal" to adjust serving sizes for unplanned meals. With three planned meals, you'll only need to measure proteins, fats and carbs for the remaining 1-3 meals as you prepare and eat them.

With all the practice you've done in the past two weeks, by now you've narrowed in and know how to hit your protein and fat goal for the day, allowing you to put more focus on tracking carbohydrates to hit your meal goals.

Summary of Week 3 Plan:
Plan 3 meals
Track Protein, fats and carbohydrates for all other meals

Jane's Food Log Examples:

Meal 1 -Breakfast (Planned Meal #1)

Food	Fat	Carb	Protein
1 eggs w/ yolk,	5g	0g	6g
1 slice cheese	6g	0g	5g
English Muffin	1g	25g	4g

Meal 2 -Morning Snack (Planned Meal #2)

Food	Fat	Carb	Protein
Protein Bar – Blueberry Cobbler	8g	24g	20g

Meal 3 – Lunch (Planned Meal #3)

Food	Fat	Carb	Protein
4oz. 93/7 beef	8g	0g	23g
Hamburger Bun	1g	28g	3g
½ cucumber	0g	4g	0g
1 tbsp. Ketchup	0g	4g	0g

Meal 4 – Afternoon Snack (Protein, Fat & Carb)

Food	Fat	Carb	Protein
Protein Shake	2g	4g	22g
Unsweetened Vanilla Alm. Milk	1g	2.5g	1g
Green Apple	0g	25g	.5g

Meal 5 - Supper (Protein, Fat & Carb)

Food	Fat	Carb	Protein
4oz 99/1 Ground Turkey	2g	0g	26g
1 tbsp. Mayonnaise & Mustard	10g	0g	0g
100g sweet potato	0g	20g	2g
Daily Total	44g	142g	112.5g

Jane hit her daily macro goal, falling within 5g on either side of her macros. Jane's Goal: F:48g, C:144g, P:108g

DAY 15

Meal 1 - (Planned Meal #1)	Fat	Carb	Protein
Meal 2 – (Planned Meal #2)	Fat	Carb	Protein
Meal 3 - (Planned Meal #3)	Fat	Carb	Protein
Meal 4 – (Protein, Fat & Carb)	Fat	Carb	Protein
Meal 5 – (Protein, Fat & Carb)	Fat	Carb	Protein
Meal 6 – (Protein, Fat & Carb)	Fat	Carb	Protein
Daily Total			

DAY 16

Meal 1 - (Planned Meal #1)	Fat	Carb	Protein
Meal 2 – (Planned Meal #2)	Fat	Carb	Protein
Meal 3 - (Planned Meal #3)	Fat	Carb	Protein
Meal 4 – (Protein, Fat & Carb)	Fat	Carb	Protein
Meal 5 – (Protein, Fat & Carb)	Fat	Carb	Protein
Meal 6 – (Protein, Fat & Carb)	Fat	Carb	Protein
Daily Total			

DAY 17

Meal 1 - (Planned Meal #1)	Fat	Carb	Protein
Meal 2 – (Planned Meal #2)	Fat	Carb	Protein
Meal 3 - (Planned Meal #3)	Fat	Carb	Protein
Meal 4 – (Protein, Fat & Carb)	Fat	Carb	Protein
Meal 5 – (Protein, Fat & Carb)	Fat	Carb	Protein
Meal 6 – (Protein, Fat & Carb)	Fat	Carb	Protein
Daily Total			

DAY 18

Meal 1 - (Planned Meal #1)	Fat	Carb	Protein
Meal 2 – (Planned Meal #2)	Fat	Carb	Protein
Meal 3 - (Planned Meal #3)	Fat	Carb	Protein
Meal 4 – (Protein, Fat & Carb)	Fat	Carb	Protein
Meal 5 – (Protein, Fat & Carb)	Fat	Carb	Protein
Meal 6 – (Protein, Fat & Carb)	Fat	Carb	Protein
Daily Total			

DAY 19

Meal 1 - (Planned Meal #1)	Fat	Carb	Protein
Meal 2 – (Planned Meal #2)	Fat	Carb	Protein
Meal 3 - (Planned Meal #3)	Fat	Carb	Protein
Meal 4 – (Protein, Fat & Carb)	Fat	Carb	Protein
Meal 5 – (Protein, Fat & Carb)	Fat	Carb	Protein
Meal 6 – (Protein, Fat & Carb)	Fat	Carb	Protein
Daily Total			

DAY 20

Meal 1 - (Planned Meal #1)	Fat	Carb	Protein
Meal 2 – (Planned Meal #2)	Fat	Carb	Protein
Meal 3 - (Planned Meal #3)	Fat	Carb	Protein
Meal 4 – (Protein, Fat & Carb)	Fat	Carb	Protein
Meal 5 – (Protein, Fat & Carb)	Fat	Carb	Protein
Meal 6 – (Protein, Fat & Carb)	Fat	Carb	Protein
Daily Total			

DAY 21

Meal 1 - (Planned Meal #1)	Fat	Carb	Protein
Meal 2 – (Planned Meal #2)	Fat	Carb	Protein
Meal 3 - (Planned Meal #3)	Fat	Carb	Protein
Meal 4 – (Protein, Fat & Carb)	Fat	Carb	Protein
Meal 5 – (Protein, Fat & Carb)	Fat	Carb	Protein
Meal 6 – (Protein, Fat & Carb)	Fat	Carb	Protein
Daily Total			

The Method: Gaining Sustainability and Flexibility

Congratulations! You have practiced and learned how to follow and track macros for your body type. This is a time to reflect on what you've learned about the foods you've tracked up to this point. Now, it comes down to practice to gain momentum. With practice ease and comfort will naturally come the more aware you become of the foods that fit into your meals the simplest.

Continue to track your macro's, become even more precise with hitting your goals, and experiment with new meals to allow yourself variety while you work to achieve results. Boredom and a bland pallet can easily sidetrack you, so I highly recommend trying new spices and incorporate foods you haven't been eating. It's also a great time to allow yourself the flexibility to add in favorite foods or treats that you may not have had for the past few weeks. Learn how you can adjust your meals so that you can have your favorite foods and stick to your macros every day. Feeling deprived is another quick way to fall off track.

Overtime, when you are closer to achieving your goals, allow yourself to attempt "eyeballing" your measurements to see how accurate you are. This will help with long term sustainability and knowing appropriate serving sizes without the need to measure.

If you fall off track, simply go back to your foundation of the "planned" meals you know you can rely on. Stay on track one meal at a time. Always aim for your macro "meal goal", it is the simplest way to stay on track.

Factoring in A Secondary Body Type

»» ———————— ««

If you do have a secondary body type, consider adjusting your macronutrients 5% -10% combining the secondary body type. (i.e. If you feel you are mainly endomorph, but also carry more fat on the hips (where a mesomorph would too), then you may want to tweak towards a mesomorph body type).

When tweaking macros, it's most often suggested to interchange your carbohydrate and fat intake as you would too per se "lean out." Lower carb/higher fat macro ratios are typically used when trying to lean out, whereas higher carb/lower fat ratios are typically used when trying to gain lean muscle mass. For example, you can drop the fat 5%-10% and increase the carb 5%-10% to tweak towards a mesomorph body type. Be sure to interchange the full amount you are taking from one macro to put into the other. Protein macros will typically remain relatively the same in both cases, around 30% of your caloric intake, give or take 5%. It's suggested to have .08 – 1g of protein per pound of body weight.

Typically, if you're at the stage of tweaking your macros to a secondary body type, you've more than likely been successful losing a portion of weight and have now found yourself at a plateau. Be patient, finding the right balance for your body is going to be a trial and error, so allow at least 1-2 weeks of consistent follow through and clean eating to know if your adjustments are working.

If you find yourself at a plateau, rather than changing your macros to a secondary body type, another great option would be to carb cycle. Carb cycling is safe, effective and in many cases, can speed up the process of fat loss.

Introducing Carb Cycling

Carb cycling can also be used to overcome a weight loss plateau or speed up your weight loss journey. I don't recommend starting this until you've completed this workbook of following the method to learning and practicing the basics of tracking macros.

What I like about carb cycling is that it's still sustainable, it can offer the advantage of getting to consume more/less of a macronutrient group, you can tailor it to your training regimen and it really works to speed up fat loss! In a nutshell, the general concept of carb cycling is to alternate your carbohydrate intake to lose body fat. High carb days offer your body fuel for intense training days, regulating hormones, and reduce muscle breakdown. Low carb days are to switch your body over to using fat for energy and train the body to burn fat as fuel in the long term.

There are a variety of carb cycles that you can follow. However, I've found Chris and Heidi Powell's (from ABC's Tv Show "Extreme Weight Loss") 5 main carb cycle schedule's to be the simplest and most effective to follow *(see next page)*.

Carb Cycle Mode	Day 1	Day 2	Day 3	Day 4	Day 5	Day 6	Day 7
Easy	low	high w/ RM	low	high w/ RM	low	high w/ RM	high w/ RM
Classic	low	high	low	high	low	high	RD
Turbo	low	low	high	low	low	high	RD
Fit	high	high	low	high	high	low	RD
Extreme	high	high	high	high	low	low	RD

(low= low carb day, high=high carb day, Reward Meal= RM (not to be eaten at supper/last meal), Reward Day= eat all the food(s) you love) "Easy" carb cycle mode suggests incorporating one reward meal for your "high carb" day.

When setting your macros for a "high carb" day, it's suggested to have 1 – 1.5 grams carbohydrates per pound of body weight and on a "low carb" day it could .5-1grams carbohydrates per pound of body weight. There is no set formula, but this is a general "macro setting" suggestion and overall an effective calculation. Your fat and protein will typically stay the same (unless you're in a temporary "lean out" phase, then you may want to interchange the fat/carb percentages). Your calorie intake will increase on your high carb days, so be sure to set your caloric intake to meet the suggested recommendations to meet your goals as I talked about in the chapter "Calculating Your Macros." A simple way to do this is to use your "daily" caloric intake as your "high carb" day, and, naturally, on "low carb" days, your calorie intake will reduce. *(i.e. Your high carb day calls for 150g carbs and 1,500kcal. You're low carb day calls for 75g carbs and 1,400kcal. Fats and Proteins remain the same).*

Frequently Asked Questions

What is the best way to meal prep? The simplest way to meal prep is to plan 2-3 meals to be consistent every day, changing it up each week if you need variety. Make some meals simple such as a bar or protein drink and fruit. For the other meals, cook enough food to have leftovers for a couple of days, so you have food to pack for workdays or quick grab.

What is the easiest way to stay on track? Knowing your "meal goal" macros so you can always select foods to hit your macros for meals. Also, always have at least two meal options that you can fall to for a "planned" meal if you don't have food prepped.

How do I stay consistent? To remain consistent, you need to know your macros for each meal. If you know this, you can easily piece together meals out of the cupboards, fridge, gas stations or fast-food restaurants. Also, allow yourself the flexibility to calculate in treats and favorite foods that aren't necessarily deemed as healthy.

How important is it to reach your macro goal? To get results within a decent timeframe, about 85% of the time. 85% of your meals should be hitting your targeted "meal goal." Falling within 5g over/under your macro goal is near perfect.

How do I add alcohol? Simply calculate the macros into your food log. Convert your calories into carbs or fats. (i.e., if the drink has 140cals, and you want to put half to carbs and half to fats, you would divide 140/2 =70. Then, divide 70/ 4 = 18g (4 calories in 1g carb) and 70/9 = 8g (9 calories in 1g fat). You could deduct 18g from carbs and 8g from fats for that 140 calorie drink.

When do you change your macro's? If you've consistently followed your macros for two weeks, out ruled that your calorie intake is correct, and have eaten "clean" foods 85% of the time with no results.

How do I measure when I cook in bulk? See the four steps on page 30.

How much sugar should I eat? 10% or less of your carbohydrate intake to reduce body fat. (i.e. Jane eats 1,439 calories, 1,439 x .10 / 4 = 36g per day for fat/weight loss)

How much can I be over/under and still get results? I recommend 5g consistently. No more than 10g 1-2 x a week.

Do you count fibrous carbohydrates? Counting them can speed up progress. However, never discredit the value of nutrition and its effects. I recommend trying both ways to see what works best for you.

Do I count saturated/unsaturated fats? A person should pay attention to fats for general health. Some saturated fats are good. It's recommended not to have more than 6% of total fat calorie intake per day. (i.e., Jane's calorie intake is 1,439 per day, it's recommended she doesn't have more than 8g. 1,439 x .05 / 9 = 7.9)

How can I incorporate carb cycling? See pages 67-68.

How do I know how much to eat for my body type? See pages 1-15 for a full break down to calculate your own.

Can I follow macros when I'm pregnant? It's recommended to increase your calories by 100 calories per trimester (i.e., add an extra 100 calories in the 1st trimester, add an extra 200 calories in the 2nd trimester, and add an extra 300 calories in the 3rd trimester). Continue to eat percentages of proteins, fats and carbs according to your body type.